MW00427007

ELIMINATION DIET JOURNAL

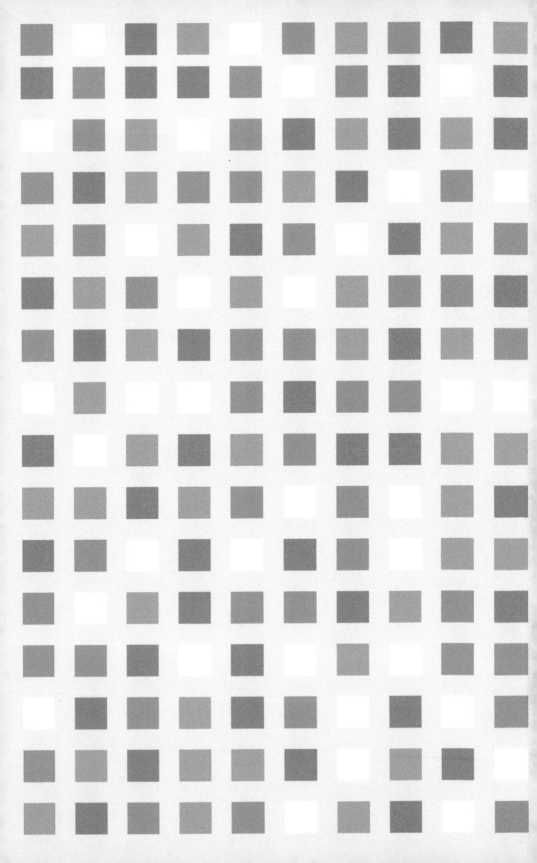

ELIMINATION DIET
JOURNAL

60-Day Symptom and Food Reintroduction Tracker

HEIDI MORETTI, MS, RD

ROCKRIDGE
PRESS

Copyright © 2022 by Rockridge Press, Emeryville, California

No part of this publication may be reproduced, stored in a retrieval system, or transmitted in any form or by any means, electronic, mechanical, photocopying, recording, scanning, or otherwise, except as permitted under Sections 107 or 108 of the 1976 United States Copyright Act, without the prior written permission of the Publisher. Requests to the Publisher for permission should be addressed to the Permissions Department, Rockridge Press, 6005 Shellmound Street, Suite 175, Emeryville, CA 94608.

Limit of Liability/Disclaimer of Warranty: The Publisher and the author make no representations or warranties with respect to the accuracy or completeness of the contents of this work and specifically disclaim all warranties, including without limitation warranties of fitness for a particular purpose. No warranty may be created or extended by sales or promotional materials. The advice and strategies contained herein may not be suitable for every situation. This work is sold with the understanding that the Publisher is not engaged in rendering medical, legal, or other professional advice or services. If professional assistance is required, the services of a competent professional person should be sought. Neither the Publisher nor the author shall be liable for damages arising herefrom. The fact that an individual, organization, or website is referred to in this work as a citation and/or potential source of further information does not mean that the author or the Publisher endorses the information the individual, organization, or website may provide or recommendations they/it may make. Further, readers should be aware that websites listed in this work may have changed or disappeared between when this work was written and when it is read.

For general information on our other products and services or to obtain technical support, please contact our Customer Care Department within the United States at (866) 744-2665, or outside the United States at (510) 253-0500.

Rockridge Press publishes its books in a variety of electronic and print formats. Some content that appears in print may not be available in electronic books, and vice versa.

TRADEMARKS: Rockridge Press and the Rockridge Press logo are trademarks or registered trademarks of Callisto Media Inc. and/or its affiliates, in the United States and other countries, and may not be used without written permission. All other trademarks are the property of their respective owners. Rockridge Press is not associated with any product or vendor mentioned in this book.

Interior and Cover Designer: Heather Krakora

Art Producer: Samantha Ulban

Editor: Rebecca Markley

Production Editor: Caroline Flanagan

Production Manager: Holly Haydash

All images used under license © iStock and Shutterstock. Author Photo Courtesy of Athena Photography.

Paperback ISBN: 978-1-64876-295-6

R0

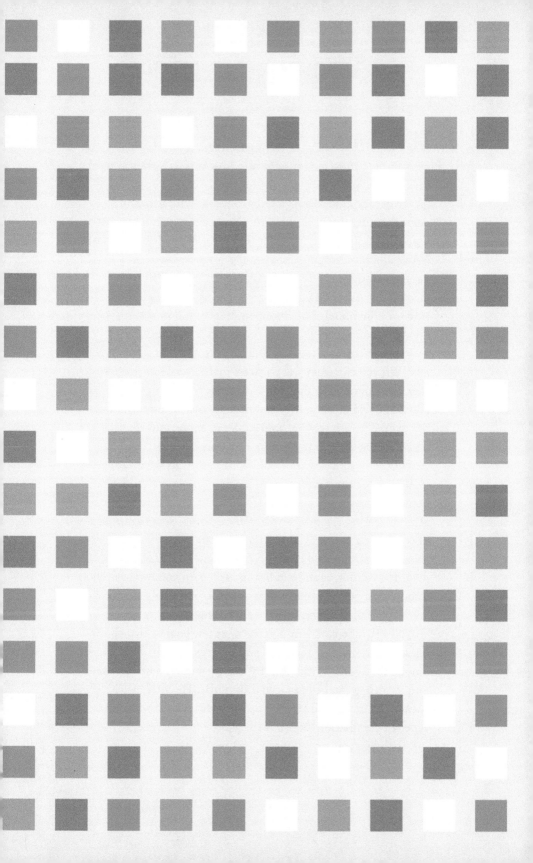

Welcome to your elimination diet journal, which is full of ways for you to gain insight into how you feel when you eat certain foods.

My background as a registered dietitian with a master's degree in nutritional science and also as a functional nutrition practitioner has given me extensive knowledge of chronic health issues like autoimmune diseases, digestive diseases, mood disorders, and fatigue conditions, and how foods are deeply related to all of these. Additionally, I have had training through the Institute for Functional Medicine about how to follow elimination diets for food sensitivities, allergies, and intolerances.

Through my own journey of following elimination diets, I can tell you that they can be transformational in a positive way. For example, by figuring out my own food triggers, I was able to get rid of brain fog, as well as digestive and skin issues. My overall health was boosted while my mood and energy improved because of my elimination diet journey.

This book is for anyone looking to figure out what foods work well for them and what foods don't. Keep in mind, this book is just as much about the foods to include as to eliminate; after all, eating is a powerful tool for healing. Some examples of conditions that an elimination diet can help with are digestive conditions, mood issues, fatigue, general malaise, skin disorders, autoimmune conditions, and pain and inflammation issues. Using this journal will be helpful for sorting out if foods are triggering or exacerbating health issues.

Make sure to read through the next few pages before jumping into the tracking section. I will be covering the differences among food sensitivities, food allergies, and food intolerances and how they can be managed differently. The root causes of these food issues will also be explored, as well as the various types of elimination diets out there.

I wish you well on your journey to wellness.

FOOD SENSITIVITIES, INTOLERANCES, AND ALLERGIES—OH MY!

You are likely here because you suspect or know that you have a food sensitivity, intolerance, or allergy, or a combination thereof. Another reason you may be here is that you realize the connection between gut health and whole-body health runs deep, and you want to gain a better understanding of how to feel better overall.

Let's take a look at the definitions of food sensitivities, food intolerances, and food allergies to help you understand these terms better, so that you can understand the differences as you begin journaling.

FOOD INTOLERANCE

Food intolerances are an inability to digest certain foods or food additives, with symptoms such as gas, bloating, abdominal pain, or reflux. They can be caused by imbalances in the microbiome, by chemical sensitivities, and by lack of digestive enzymes.

FOOD SENSITIVITY

Food sensitivities are caused by an immune reaction to foods, with symptoms similar to those of food intolerances. However, this type of reaction can cause moderate changes in the whole body and mind, too. Some examples include skin reactions, mood swings, brain fog, and muscle aches, among others. A challenging part of identifying food sensitivities is that it can take up to three to four days after ingesting a food to see a reaction, making them difficult to pinpoint.

FOOD ALLERGY

A true food allergy involves a more severe immune reaction to a food because it causes an immunoglobulin E antibody response. True food allergies also usually happen more quickly than food sensitivities. Symptoms of food allergies can include rashes, difficulties breathing, digestive symptoms, hives, fatigue, and more.

COMMON UNDERLYING CONDITIONS

Food allergies, sensitivities, or intolerances are typically related to other health conditions. The following list of disorders is only a partial list of possible reasons that you may have problems with various foods.

Irritable bowel syndrome (IBS): If you have irritable bowel syndrome, odds are you also have an allergy, sensitivity, or intolerance to one or more foods. Not surprisingly, IBS is rooted in many causes and is a catch-all term for people who have unexplained abdominal pain and abnormal bowel movements on a frequent basis.

Imbalanced microbiome: Your microbiome consists of the living organisms in your gut. These bacteria and other coinhabitants often determine how your body responds to food. An imbalanced microbiome is often the result of eating processed foods and food additives.

Autoimmune conditions: Although celiac disease has received a lot of attention recently, research shows that many people with autoimmune diseases also suffer from immune-related food allergies and intolerances.

Inadequate digestive enzymes: A lack of adequate digestive enzymes can be a trigger for food intolerances and sensitivities. Although there is no way to officially test for digestive enzymes, many people find out they are lacking enzymes when they eat certain foods. A good example of this is lactose intolerance in people who lack adequate lactase enzymes.

Inflammation: When the lining of your gut is inflamed, the condition of your gut is imbalanced and may cause a reduction in food tolerance. Gut inflammation can be caused by processed foods or inflammatory bowel diseases, like ulcerative colitis or Crohn's disease.

Stress: Being stressed alters gut mobility, reduces the production of digestive enzymes, and decreases the health of the microbiome, too.

Previous abdominal surgeries: Abdominal surgeries can often result in digestive issues. Sometimes there's a reduction in stomach acid production, which is what helps break down otherwise allergic food proteins. Also, these surgeries often change the ability to have normal bowel movements, which can cause new food intolerances due to bacterial overgrowth.

Sensitivity? Or Typical Digestion?

You may be wondering how to sort out whether you are having a food sensitivity reaction or having typical digestion with some types of foods. Typical digestion with foods like onions, garlic, hot peppers, beans, lentils, and vegetables in the broccoli family can result in temporary gas, bloating, and reflux. Almost everyone has these reactions to these foods unless the food is prepared properly or digestive enzymes are taken when eating them.

There are some simple ways to help deal with typical digestion symptoms. For example, using Beano, which is a single-enzyme supplement, helps break down the fibers that cause gas. Other types of enzyme supplements on the market today are broader spectrum and may help you digest these challenging foods better than a single-enzyme supplement. Remember, our bodies make many types of digestive enzymes to break down foods, so it makes sense to find one that has a variety of types of enzymes.

Another example of typical digestive upset occurs when you suddenly and substantially increase the quantity of fibrous foods like oats, quinoa, fruits, or vegetables in your diet. Gas and bloating may occur because the gut doesn't have time to increase its enzyme production, and you may develop food intolerance symptoms as a result.

Food sensitivity reactions can cause gas and bloating, too, but these symptoms will linger longer than typical digestive reactions, which should last for only a few hours after eating the trigger food. Also, in the case of a food sensitivity, other symptoms, such as body aches, brain fog, mood changes, or skin conditions, may appear over the next few days.

You can reduce typical food reactions by soaking, sprouting, fermenting, and cooking the trigger foods. These steps not only help you digest the foods better but also increase nutritional value and help create a healthier microbiome. More good news is that by following an elimination diet, you may heal your gut so that you make more digestive enzymes. For example, I used to have a food intolerance to raw broccoli. After following the elimination diet, I can now tolerate large amounts of raw broccoli!

WHY DO AN ELIMINATION DIET?

An elimination diet is a type of eating plan that removes foods, over a short period of time, that are common causes of adverse food reactions. This elimination phase is followed by an important phase called the challenge period, when foods are reintroduced one by one to see if they create health problems.

Many people are surprised to find out that an elimination diet is actually the gold standard of determining food sensitivities, allergies, and intolerances. Blood work, although useful, is not as accurate for these conditions as we would hope it could be at this point. Additionally, the cost of food sensitivity and allergy testing is high, and results may not be as accurate as those you will get from following an elimination diet.

There are also five surprising reasons that may inspire you to do an elimination diet:

1. **Your skin health may improve.** Food reactions can be a sneaky cause of acne, dry patches, eczema, dull skin, reddened skin, and other adverse skin conditions.

2. **The energy you gain might surprise you.** If you are constantly reacting to food, it makes you tired. By eliminating a food trigger, you may find that your energy levels get a substantial boost.

3. **Your brain may get a needed boost.** By eliminating trigger foods, you may feel more focused, calm, and happy.

4. **Joint aches and pains may dissipate.** Food reactions are a big cause of inflammation, so when you eliminate these triggers, your joints and body may feel a lot better, too.

5. **You may enjoy a lifelong reset of better eating.** Many people who try an elimination diet are surprised to find out that their eating patterns change for the better in the long term as they become naturally more self-aware of how they respond to certain foods.

Types of Elimination Diets

There are five common types of elimination diets, with the gold standard being the Elimination Diet. It's important for you to work with your healthcare provider to determine the best approach for you.

The Elimination Diet involves eliminating the most common food allergens and processed foods. These include gluten, dairy, soy, corn, eggs, shellfish, peanuts, tree nuts, processed sugars, and processed snacks and meals. This is the plan that this journal covers in depth.

Low-FODMAP is a meal plan that minimizes fermentable carbohydrate foods, such as wheat, most dairy, some fruits, vegetables, sugar, and some other grains. Typically, this meal plan is used to uncover IBS or bacterial overgrowth in the small intestine but can miss other food sensitivities that aren't low-FODMAP (fermentable oligosaccharides, disaccharides, monosaccharides, and polyols).

GAPS is the Gut and Psychology Syndrome (GAPS) diet, used for people struggling with autism, mood disorders, and autoimmune disorders. It focuses on healing the gut and enhancing the microbiome. This diet eliminates all dairy, legumes, and grains, as well as low-nutrient-density foods, but includes all high-nutrient-density foods.

The LEAP Diet is based on foods that the body mounts an inflammation response to, so it is highly individualized for each person. The downsides are that this elimination diet can take a long time, and the testing is more expensive than for the standard elimination diet.

A Simple Elimination Diet eliminates only one or two foods at a time, usually gluten or dairy, which are the most common food triggers for food sensitivities, food intolerance, and food allergies. Although easiest to follow, this diet often does not pinpoint all the food sensitivities and intolerances a person might have.

THE ELIMINATION DIET
IN THREE PHASES

This section describes the phases of the elimination diet to help you know what to expect. Phase 1 typically takes about a week. I recommend that you spend four weeks each on both Phase 2 and Phase 3.

PHASE 1: PREPARING (1 WEEK)

The first step in an elimination diet is preparation. You will need to assess if you have the time to follow through with an eight-week plan. For example, do not try to do this plan if you are traveling or undergoing medical procedures or currently have a high level of stress in your life.

Use this week to grocery shop, develop a menu, and clear your calendar for the next couple of months to allow your focus to stay on healing your gut. You should also evaluate with your healthcare provider which foods to remove so that you feel comfortable about moving forward with the diet. Use the first three or four days of journal entries to track your current way of eating so that you can see your full progression at the end of the 60 days.

PHASE 2: ELIMINATION (4 WEEKS)

Phase 2 is when you will eliminate all suspected trigger foods. Remember, however, that the foods you keep are just as important as the foods you remove. In order to be successful, you will need to stick with the plan for the whole month, so you need foods that will heal your gut but that are also satisfying and delicious. If you accidentally eat an excluded food on the list one time, don't despair—just get right back on track. Usually, you don't need to start over unless the target food is eaten multiple times, but make sure to note when and how much you ate and how you feel as part of that day's journal entry.

Also be aware that during the first week of the elimination diet, you may feel a bit worse before you feel better. This is called a healing reaction, which means that your body may be releasing toxins that have built up. You may also feel some distress due to withdrawal as you taper your caffeine and sugar intake. These symptoms are usually mild but can include some body aches, digestive distress, mood changes, and even fatigue. Make sure to stay the course through this, and you will most likely be rewarded with a dramatic improvement in how you feel shortly thereafter.

═ PHASE 3: REINTRODUCTION (4 WEEKS) ═

Phase 3 is just as important as phase 2 because this is when you figure out which foods are your trigger foods. It can feel slow, and you may be impatient at this point to add back all the eliminated foods. However, it's imperative that you patiently add foods back one at a time so your body can tell you what you need to know. This happens because after the elimination of a food, your body will be highly sensitized when any offending food is reintroduced.

During this phase, reintroduce a single food for three consecutive days, and monitor your symptoms using the food journal. If you have any reaction to the reintroduced food, do not eat any more of that food, and wait another two days before reintroducing the next target food. If you have no reaction, you can simply add the next food after day 3 of reintroduction, and you won't need to remove that food again. You will want to continue this process for another four weeks or so, depending on how you are feeling and how many foods you removed. Here are some other rules for success during this period:

→ Reintroduce the single-ingredient food you missed the most first.
→ Make sure to eat at least two full servings of the reintroduced food throughout the day; a serving would be 5 to 10 crackers, 1 ounce of cheese, 1 cup of milk, etc.
→ Avoid foods that tend to be combined with other ingredients. For example, bread and buns, or pizza. Instead, add back either wheat farina or a simple soda cracker. Bread has many additives and other possible allergens, so you may not get a clear picture of your triggers if you don't go ingredient by ingredient.
→ Make sure to add the reintroduced food for three full days. If this food causes a symptom, you will need to remove it throughout the reintroduction phase and likely keep it out of your diet indefinitely to keep you healthy. Remember to wait two days before reintroducing the next food.

TIPS FOR SUCCESS

Although the elimination diet can be very rewarding, it can also be frustrating. Planning meals ahead of time and having foods on hand that fit your diet are keys to success.

MEAL PLANNING

Don't skimp on eating. You need to make sure you are full and satisfied for a few reasons: to get adequate nutrients for gut healing, to minimize any discomfort, and to help keep you from straying from the plan.

Find substitutes. Brainstorm the usual foods you eat, and write them down. Then create a list of substitutes that you can have instead of these items. For example, if you like having burgers, make your burgers "protein style" by wrapping them in lettuce instead of a bun.

Choose simple combinations. Make a list of the foods you enjoy the most based on the ideas you came up with earlier. Simple is almost always the way to go on an elimination diet: choose your protein, veggies, a starch, a fat, and spices for each meal. For example, salmon with assorted veggies sautéed with extra-virgin olive oil, basil, and garlic over sweet potatoes.

SHOPPING SHORTCUTS

Shop fresh. Stick to the perimeter of the grocery store to find whole foods like produce, healthy oils, and dry goods.

Read labels carefully. Make sure to read food labels carefully and look for any ingredients likely to cause sensitivities or allergic responses. Specifically, read the labels of condiments, since they often contain a lot of additives.

Don't shop when hungry. Make sure to eat before shopping so that you don't buy extra treats or foods that aren't on your food list.

Buy organic when possible. Organic produce and products contain fewer additives and chemicals that your body may react to.

Precut veggies. Buy precut veggies to save yourself time and effort.

Other Lifestyle Tips

Even though this book is primarily focused on diet, you will want to track other lifestyle habits that affect your progress, such as sleep, sun exposure, stress, exercise, and social activities.

Sleep: Note in your journal if your sleep is "very good," "good," "suboptimal," or "poor." "Very good" sleep is at least 6 to 8 hours of restful sleep, and "good" sleep is restful with brief periods of waking. A "suboptimal" sleep is broken sleep, leading to mild periods of fatigue during the day, and "poor" sleep impairs your day-to-day activities, resulting in forgetfulness and exhaustion. The other tips on this list will help with sleep quality.

Sun exposure: Exposure to early and midday sunlight plays an important role in keeping your gut healthy and improving your sleep cycles. Track the amount of time you spend outside each day in your journal to help you identify patterns.

Stress: Track your stress levels, indicating if you are having high, moderate, low, or no stress. Take time to relax, meditate, do yoga, and listen to relaxing music to help minimize your stress levels.

Exercise: Physical activity helps with digestion, sleep, and stress levels. Why not also get some sun exposure while you are at it? Use your lunchtime and breaks at work as times to get in quick walks or a stretch.

Social activities: Spend time with supportive friends and family to help you feel your best. Just make sure that when you gather, you inform them of your elimination diet needs and have suitable dishes on hand if your social activities include a meal.

Dietary supplements: Adding an all-natural, broad-spectrum vitamin with minerals supplement can be helpful in speeding up the healing of the gut when going through the elimination diet. A few brands to look for include Thorne Research, Seeking Health, Klaire Labs, and Pure Encapsulations. Adding a broad-spectrum digestive enzyme supplement at meals can be very beneficial, too. I particularly like Seeking Health Digestion Intensive and Pure Encapsulations Digestive Enzymes, which are both Good Manufacturing Practices–certified and broad spectrum to help digest many types of foods.

USING THE JOURNAL

This journal is designed to be very straightforward, but there are a couple of important things to know before you get going. Please note that it is a good idea to keep the journal for a few days before you begin the elimination diet so that you can have a baseline record of your starting point.

TRACKING YOUR FOOD "RESPONSE"

The response sections are there to help you record any changes in your physical and mental health, your eating habits, where you are eating, and any other pertinent information related to the periods before or after your mealtimes.

Be mindful of things like stomachache, belching, sour stomach, bloating, changes in bowel movements, abdominal pain, mental focus, mood changes, menstrual cycle changes (if applicable), and energy levels. Make sure to make note of any positive changes you are noticing as well.

For example, if you feel really fatigued after lunch, make note of it in your journal. If you notice that your stomach hurts, make sure to note if you ate too quickly, didn't chew your food well, or were stressed at the time you ate the meal. If you feel bloating, note if you are eating a new food or a large quantity of a food. Also take note of how the food was prepared. For instance, if you are eating black beans, were they soaked for at least 12 hours and rinsed? Did you include a digestive enzyme supplement at the time?

Finally, in the mornings, note how well you slept the night before because the foods you ate the previous day can impact sleep quality.

Although many factors will affect how you feel after you eat, this careful journaling will help you see patterns in how your habits and diet are affecting how you feel.

BRISTOL STOOL CHART

The Bristol stool chart will help you become familiar with your bowel movement patterns and how to make note of changes in your stools throughout the elimination diet. Bowel movements, which are driven by the foods you eat, are critical to a healthy body and mind because they remove harmful waste from the body.

It's also a good idea to make note of the color of your stool. A normal bowel movement will be medium to dark brown. Light or pasty-colored stools, as well as black or red stools (unless you are eating beets or taking iron), are a sign you need to seek help from your healthcare provider.

TYPE	DESCRIPTION
1-severe constipation	Separate, hard lumps of stool that are hard to pass
2-mild constipation	Formed, sausage-shaped, but lumpy and somewhat hard to pass
3-normal	Sausage-shaped with cracks on the surface, easy to pass
4-normal	Smooth, snakelike, and soft, easy to pass
5-lacking fiber	Blobs of stool that have clear-cut edges, pass too quickly
6-mild diarrhea	Mushy consistency with ragged edges, passes too quickly, often more than once a day
7-severe diarrhea	Liquid consistency multiple times a day

DATE: _January 7_   PHASE: ①   2   3

BREAKFAST / TIME _8:35 A.M._	RESPONSE
Oatmeal	Upset stomach but still hungry.
Strawberries	

LUNCH / TIME _1:15 P.M._	RESPONSE
Chicken breast	Upset stomach gone. Feel full.
Green beans	
Apple	

DINNER / TIME _6:30 P.M._	RESPONSE
Black bean burger on lettuce wrap	
Jicama fries	

SNACKS / BEVERAGES	RESPONSE
Green tea	

REINTRODUCED FOOD (PHASE 3 ONLY): _____

BOWEL MOVEMENTS		
TIME	**TYPE**	**NOTES**
8:45 a.m.	2	Slightly hard to pass. Still felt constipated.

VITAMIN / MEDICATION	DOSAGE	TIME
Multivitamin	1 pill	8 a.m.

H2O* 🖋 🖋 🖋 🖋 🖋 💧 💧 💧 💧 💧

SLEEP LAST NIGHT: 6 hrs. **BEDTIME:** 11:30 p.m.

☐ Very Good   ☐ Good   ☒ Suboptimal   ☐ Poor

TODAY'S OVERALL MOOD: 1 2 3 ④ 5   (HAPPIEST)

TODAY'S OVERALL STRESS: 1 ② 3 4 5   (MOST STRESSED)

ADDITIONAL NOTES:	Ran 2 miles, felt great.
Physical Activity?	
Other Symptoms?	Have work birthday celebration tomorrow so taking my own sweet treat (apples and dip).
Infections?	
Menstrual Cycle?	
Vitals?	
Weight?	
Other Habits Being Tracked?	
Special Events?	

*10 ounces per drop

ELIMINATION CHECK-IN

SYMPTOM ASSESSMENT

0=No issues; 1=Light; 2=Mild; 3=Extreme

SYMPTOM	BEFORE ELIMINATION DIET	AFTER ELIMINATION DIET
Aches/pains		
Anxiety		
Asthma		
Brain fog		
Chronic sinus drainage		
Cold extremities		
Congestion		
Depression		
Digestive issues (bloating, gas, upset stomach)		
Fatigue		
Headaches/migraines		
Inflammation		
Skin irritation		
Sleep		
Stress		
Weight gain/loss		
Other:		
Other:		
Other:		
Other:		
Other:		

REINTRODUCTION CHECK-IN

REINTRODUCED FOOD/SERVING SIZE	DATE

DATE:_____   PHASE: 1   2   3

BREAKFAST / TIME_____	RESPONSE

LUNCH / TIME_____	RESPONSE

DINNER / TIME_____	RESPONSE

SNACKS / BEVERAGES	RESPONSE

REINTRODUCED FOOD (PHASE 3 ONLY): _____
BOWEL MOVEMENTS

VITAMIN / MEDICATION	DOSAGE	TIME

H2O* ⬦ ⬦ ⬦ ⬦ ⬦ ⬦ ⬦ ⬦ ⬦ ⬦

SLEEP LAST NIGHT: _____ Hrs. **BEDTIME:** _____

☐ Very Good   ☐ Good   ☐ Suboptimal   ☐ Poor

TODAY'S OVERALL MOOD: 1 2 3 4 5 (HAPPIEST)

TODAY'S OVERALL STRESS: 1 2 3 4 5 (MOST STRESSED)

ADDITIONAL NOTES:

Physical Activity?

Other Symptoms?

Infections?

Menstrual Cycle?

Vitals?

Weight?

Other Habits Being Tracked?

Special Events?

*10 ounces per drop

21

DATE:_____ PHASE: 1   2   3

BREAKFAST / TIME _____	RESPONSE

LUNCH / TIME _____	RESPONSE

DINNER / TIME _____	RESPONSE

SNACKS / BEVERAGES	RESPONSE

REINTRODUCED FOOD (PHASE 3 ONLY): _____

BOWEL MOVEMENTS		
TIME	**TYPE**	**NOTES**

VITAMIN / MEDICATION	DOSAGE	TIME

H2O* ◊ ◊ ◊ ◊ ◊ ◊ ◊ ◊ ◊ ◊

SLEEP LAST NIGHT: _____ Hrs. **BEDTIME:** _____

☐ Very Good   ☐ Good   ☐ Suboptimal   ☐ Poor

TODAY'S OVERALL MOOD: 1 2 3 4 5 (HAPPIEST)

TODAY'S OVERALL STRESS: 1 2 3 4 5 (MOST STRESSED)

ADDITIONAL NOTES:

Physical Activity?

Other Symptoms?

Infections?

Menstrual Cycle?

Vitals?

Weight?

Other Habits Being Tracked?

Special Events?

*10 ounces per drop

DATE:_____ PHASE: 1   2   3

BREAKFAST / TIME_____	RESPONSE

LUNCH / TIME_____	RESPONSE

DINNER / TIME_____	RESPONSE

SNACKS / BEVERAGES	RESPONSE

REINTRODUCED FOOD (PHASE 3 ONLY): _____

BOWEL MOVEMENTS		
TIME	TYPE	NOTES

VITAMIN / MEDICATION	DOSAGE	TIME

H2O*   ◌   ◌   ◌   ◌   ◌   ◌   ◌   ◌   ◌   ◌

SLEEP LAST NIGHT: _____ Hrs. **BEDTIME:** _____

☐ Very Good   ☐ Good   ☐ Suboptimal   ☐ Poor

TODAY'S OVERALL MOOD: 1 2 3 4 5 (HAPPIEST)

TODAY'S OVERALL STRESS: 1 2 3 4 5 (MOST STRESSED)

ADDITIONAL NOTES:

Physical Activity?

Other Symptoms?

Infections?

Menstrual Cycle?

Vitals?

Weight?

Other Habits Being Tracked?

Special Events?

*10 ounces per drop

DATE:_____ PHASE: 1   2   3

BREAKFAST / TIME_____	RESPONSE

LUNCH / TIME_____	RESPONSE

DINNER / TIME_____	RESPONSE

SNACKS / BEVERAGES	RESPONSE

REINTRODUCED FOOD (PHASE 3 ONLY): _____

BOWEL MOVEMENTS

TIME	TYPE	NOTES

VITAMIN / MEDICATION	DOSAGE	TIME

H2O* ⬠ ⬠ ⬠ ⬠ ⬠ ⬠ ⬠ ⬠ ⬠ ⬠

SLEEP LAST NIGHT: _____ Hrs. **BEDTIME:** _____

☐ Very Good ☐ Good ☐ Suboptimal ☐ Poor

TODAY'S OVERALL MOOD: 1 2 3 4 5 (HAPPIEST)

TODAY'S OVERALL STRESS: 1 2 3 4 5 (MOST STRESSED)

ADDITIONAL NOTES:

Physical Activity?

Other Symptoms?

Infections?

Menstrual Cycle?

Vitals?

Weight?

Other Habits Being Tracked?

Special Events?

*10 ounces per drop

27

DATE:_____ PHASE: 1   2   3

BREAKFAST / TIME_____	RESPONSE

LUNCH / TIME_____	RESPONSE

DINNER / TIME_____	RESPONSE

SNACKS / BEVERAGES	RESPONSE

REINTRODUCED FOOD (PHASE 3 ONLY): _____

BOWEL MOVEMENTS		
TIME	TYPE	NOTES

VITAMIN / MEDICATION	DOSAGE	TIME

H2O* ○ ○ ○ ○ ○ ○ ○ ○ ○ ○

SLEEP LAST NIGHT: _____ Hrs. **BEDTIME:** _____

☐ Very Good   ☐ Good   ☐ Suboptimal   ☐ Poor

TODAY'S OVERALL MOOD: 1 2 3 4 5 (HAPPIEST)

TODAY'S OVERALL STRESS: 1 2 3 4 5 (MOST STRESSED)

ADDITIONAL NOTES:

Physical Activity?

Other Symptoms?

Infections?

Menstrual Cycle?

Vitals?

Weight?

Other Habits Being
Tracked?

Special Events?

*10 ounces per drop

DATE:_____ PHASE: 1   2   3

BREAKFAST / TIME_____	RESPONSE

LUNCH / TIME_____	RESPONSE

DINNER / TIME_____	RESPONSE

SNACKS / BEVERAGES	RESPONSE

REINTRODUCED FOOD (PHASE 3 ONLY): _____

BOWEL MOVEMENTS		
TIME	TYPE	NOTES

VITAMIN / MEDICATION	DOSAGE	TIME

H2O* ⬧ ⬧ ⬧ ⬧ ⬧ ⬧ ⬧ ⬧ ⬧ ⬧

SLEEP LAST NIGHT: _____ Hrs. **BEDTIME:** _____

☐ Very Good ☐ Good ☐ Suboptimal ☐ Poor

TODAY'S OVERALL MOOD: 1 2 3 4 5 (HAPPIEST)

TODAY'S OVERALL STRESS: 1 2 3 4 5 (MOST STRESSED)

ADDITIONAL NOTES:

Physical Activity?

Other Symptoms?

Infections?

Menstrual Cycle?

Vitals?

Weight?

Other Habits Being Tracked?

Special Events?

*10 ounces per drop

DATE:_____ PHASE: 1   2   3

BREAKFAST / TIME_____	RESPONSE

LUNCH / TIME_____	RESPONSE

DINNER / TIME_____	RESPONSE

SNACKS / BEVERAGES	RESPONSE

REINTRODUCED FOOD (PHASE 3 ONLY): _____

BOWEL MOVEMENTS		
TIME	TYPE	NOTES

VITAMIN / MEDICATION	DOSAGE	TIME

H2O* ⬦ ⬦ ⬦ ⬦ ⬦ ⬦ ⬦ ⬦ ⬦ ⬦

SLEEP LAST NIGHT: _____ Hrs. **BEDTIME:** _____

☐ Very Good ☐ Good ☐ Suboptimal ☐ Poor

TODAY'S OVERALL MOOD: 1 2 3 4 5 (HAPPIEST)

TODAY'S OVERALL STRESS: 1 2 3 4 5 (MOST STRESSED)

ADDITIONAL NOTES:	
Physical Activity?	
Other Symptoms?	
Infections?	
Menstrual Cycle?	
Vitals?	
Weight?	
Other Habits Being Tracked?	
Special Events?	

*10 ounces per drop

DATE:_____   PHASE: 1   2   3

BREAKFAST / TIME_____	RESPONSE

LUNCH / TIME_____	RESPONSE

DINNER / TIME_____	RESPONSE

SNACKS / BEVERAGES	RESPONSE

REINTRODUCED FOOD (PHASE 3 ONLY): _____

BOWEL MOVEMENTS		
TIME	**TYPE**	**NOTES**

VITAMIN / MEDICATION	DOSAGE	TIME

H2O* ⬡ ⬡ ⬡ ⬡ ⬡ ⬡ ⬡ ⬡ ⬡ ⬡

SLEEP LAST NIGHT: _____ Hrs. **BEDTIME:** _____

☐ Very Good   ☐ Good   ☐ Suboptimal   ☐ Poor

TODAY'S OVERALL MOOD: 1 2 3 4 5 (HAPPIEST)

TODAY'S OVERALL STRESS: 1 2 3 4 5 (MOST STRESSED)

ADDITIONAL NOTES:

Physical Activity?

Other Symptoms?

Infections?

Menstrual Cycle?

Vitals?

Weight?

Other Habits Being Tracked?

Special Events?

*10 ounces per drop

DATE:_____   PHASE: 1   2   3

BREAKFAST / TIME_____	RESPONSE

LUNCH / TIME_____	RESPONSE

DINNER / TIME_____	RESPONSE

SNACKS / BEVERAGES	RESPONSE

REINTRODUCED FOOD (PHASE 3 ONLY): _____

BOWEL MOVEMENTS		
TIME	TYPE	NOTES

VITAMIN / MEDICATION	DOSAGE	TIME

H2O* ⬦ ⬦ ⬦ ⬦ ⬦ ⬦ ⬦ ⬦ ⬦ ⬦

SLEEP LAST NIGHT: _____ Hrs. **BEDTIME:** _____

☐ Very Good ☐ Good ☐ Suboptimal ☐ Poor

TODAY'S OVERALL MOOD: 1 2 3 4 5 (HAPPIEST)

TODAY'S OVERALL STRESS: 1 2 3 4 5 (MOST STRESSED)

ADDITIONAL NOTES:

Physical Activity?

Other Symptoms?

Infections?

Menstrual Cycle?

Vitals?

Weight?

Other Habits Being Tracked?

Special Events?

*10 ounces per drop

DATE:_____   PHASE: 1   2   3

BREAKFAST / TIME_____	RESPONSE

LUNCH / TIME_____	RESPONSE

DINNER / TIME_____	RESPONSE

SNACKS / BEVERAGES	RESPONSE

REINTRODUCED FOOD (PHASE 3 ONLY): _____

BOWEL MOVEMENTS		
TIME	**TYPE**	**NOTES**

VITAMIN / MEDICATION	DOSAGE	TIME

H2O* ⬭ ⬭ ⬭ ⬭ ⬭ ⬭ ⬭ ⬭ ⬭ ⬭

SLEEP LAST NIGHT: _____ Hrs. **BEDTIME:** _____

☐ Very Good   ☐ Good   ☐ Suboptimal   ☐ Poor

TODAY'S OVERALL MOOD: 1 2 3 4 5 (HAPPIEST)

TODAY'S OVERALL STRESS: 1 2 3 4 5 (MOST STRESSED)

ADDITIONAL NOTES:

Physical Activity?

Other Symptoms?

Infections?

Menstrual Cycle?

Vitals?

Weight?

Other Habits Being Tracked?

Special Events?

*10 ounces per drop

DATE:_____   PHASE: 1   2   3

BREAKFAST / TIME_____	RESPONSE

LUNCH / TIME_____	RESPONSE

DINNER / TIME_____	RESPONSE

SNACKS / BEVERAGES	RESPONSE

REINTRODUCED FOOD (PHASE 3 ONLY): _____

BOWEL MOVEMENTS

TIME	TYPE	NOTES

VITAMIN / MEDICATION	DOSAGE	TIME

H2O* ⬦ ⬦ ⬦ ⬦ ⬦ ⬦ ⬦ ⬦ ⬦ ⬦

SLEEP LAST NIGHT: _____ Hrs. **BEDTIME:** _____

☐ Very Good   ☐ Good   ☐ Suboptimal   ☐ Poor

TODAY'S OVERALL MOOD: 1 2 3 4 5 (HAPPIEST)

TODAY'S OVERALL STRESS: 1 2 3 4 5 (MOST STRESSED)

ADDITIONAL NOTES:

Physical Activity?

Other Symptoms?

Infections?

Menstrual Cycle?

Vitals?

Weight?

Other Habits Being Tracked?

Special Events?

*10 ounces per drop

DATE:_____ PHASE: 1   2   3

BREAKFAST / TIME_____	RESPONSE

LUNCH / TIME_____	RESPONSE

DINNER / TIME_____	RESPONSE

SNACKS / BEVERAGES	RESPONSE

REINTRODUCED FOOD (PHASE 3 ONLY): _____

BOWEL MOVEMENTS		
TIME	TYPE	NOTES

VITAMIN / MEDICATION	DOSAGE	TIME

H2O* 　 ◊　 ◊　 ◊　 ◊　 ◊　 ◊　 ◊　 ◊　 ◊　 ◊

SLEEP LAST NIGHT: _____ Hrs. **BEDTIME:** _____

☐ Very Good ☐ Good ☐ Suboptimal ☐ Poor

TODAY'S OVERALL MOOD: 1 2 3 4 5 (HAPPIEST)

TODAY'S OVERALL STRESS: 1 2 3 4 5 (MOST STRESSED)

ADDITIONAL NOTES:

Physical Activity?

Other Symptoms?

Infections?

Menstrual Cycle?

Vitals?

Weight?

Other Habits Being Tracked?

Special Events?

*10 ounces per drop

DATE:_____ PHASE: 1   2   3

BREAKFAST / TIME_____	RESPONSE

LUNCH / TIME_____	RESPONSE

DINNER / TIME_____	RESPONSE

SNACKS / BEVERAGES	RESPONSE

REINTRODUCED FOOD (PHASE 3 ONLY): _____

BOWEL MOVEMENTS		
TIME	TYPE	NOTES

VITAMIN / MEDICATION	DOSAGE	TIME

H2O* ○ ○ ○ ○ ○ ○ ○ ○ ○ ○

SLEEP LAST NIGHT: _____ Hrs. **BEDTIME:** _____

☐ Very Good ☐ Good ☐ Suboptimal ☐ Poor

TODAY'S OVERALL MOOD: 1 2 3 4 5 (HAPPIEST)

TODAY'S OVERALL STRESS: 1 2 3 4 5 (MOST STRESSED)

ADDITIONAL NOTES:

Physical Activity?

Other Symptoms?

Infections?

Menstrual Cycle?

Vitals?

Weight?

Other Habits Being
Tracked?

Special Events?

*10 ounces per drop

DATE:_____   PHASE: 1   2   3

BREAKFAST / TIME_____	RESPONSE

LUNCH / TIME_____	RESPONSE

DINNER / TIME_____	RESPONSE

SNACKS / BEVERAGES	RESPONSE

REINTRODUCED FOOD (PHASE 3 ONLY): _____

BOWEL MOVEMENTS		
TIME	TYPE	NOTES

VITAMIN / MEDICATION	DOSAGE	TIME

H2O* ⬦ ⬦ ⬦ ⬦ ⬦ ⬦ ⬦ ⬦ ⬦ ⬦

SLEEP LAST NIGHT: _____ Hrs. **BEDTIME:** _____

☐ Very Good   ☐ Good   ☐ Suboptimal   ☐ Poor

TODAY'S OVERALL MOOD: 1 2 3 4 5 (HAPPIEST)

TODAY'S OVERALL STRESS: 1 2 3 4 5 (MOST STRESSED)

ADDITIONAL NOTES:	
Physical Activity?	
Other Symptoms?	
Infections?	
Menstrual Cycle?	
Vitals?	
Weight?	
Other Habits Being Tracked?	
Special Events?	

*10 ounces per drop

DATE:_____ PHASE: 1   2   3

BREAKFAST / TIME_____	RESPONSE

LUNCH / TIME_____	RESPONSE

DINNER / TIME_____	RESPONSE

SNACKS / BEVERAGES	RESPONSE

REINTRODUCED FOOD (PHASE 3 ONLY): _____

BOWEL MOVEMENTS

TIME	TYPE	NOTES

VITAMIN / MEDICATION	DOSAGE	TIME

H2O* ○ ○ ○ ○ ○ ○ ○ ○ ○ ○

SLEEP LAST NIGHT: _____ Hrs. **BEDTIME:** _____

☐ Very Good   ☐ Good   ☐ Suboptimal   ☐ Poor

TODAY'S OVERALL MOOD: 1 2 3 4 5 (HAPPIEST)

TODAY'S OVERALL STRESS: 1 2 3 4 5 (MOST STRESSED)

ADDITIONAL NOTES:

Physical Activity?

Other Symptoms?

Infections?

Menstrual Cycle?

Vitals?

Weight?

Other Habits Being Tracked?

Special Events?

*10 ounces per drop

49

DATE:_____ PHASE: 1   2   3

BREAKFAST / TIME_____	RESPONSE

LUNCH / TIME_____	RESPONSE

DINNER / TIME_____	RESPONSE

SNACKS / BEVERAGES	RESPONSE

REINTRODUCED FOOD (PHASE 3 ONLY): _____

BOWEL MOVEMENTS

TIME	TYPE	NOTES

VITAMIN / MEDICATION	DOSAGE	TIME

H2O* ◌   ◌   ◌   ◌   ◌   ◌   ◌   ◌   ◌   ◌

SLEEP LAST NIGHT: _____ Hrs. **BEDTIME:** _____

☐ Very Good   ☐ Good   ☐ Suboptimal   ☐ Poor

TODAY'S OVERALL MOOD: 1 2 3 4 5 (HAPPIEST)

TODAY'S OVERALL STRESS: 1 2 3 4 5 (MOST STRESSED)

ADDITIONAL NOTES:

Physical Activity?

Other Symptoms?

Infections?

Menstrual Cycle?

Vitals?

Weight?

Other Habits Being
Tracked?

Special Events?

*10 ounces per drop

51

DATE:_____   PHASE: 1   2   3

BREAKFAST / TIME_____	RESPONSE

LUNCH / TIME_____	RESPONSE

DINNER / TIME_____	RESPONSE

SNACKS / BEVERAGES	RESPONSE

REINTRODUCED FOOD (PHASE 3 ONLY): _____

BOWEL MOVEMENTS		
TIME	TYPE	NOTES

VITAMIN / MEDICATION	DOSAGE	TIME

H2O* ⬦ ⬦ ⬦ ⬦ ⬦ ⬦ ⬦ ⬦ ⬦ ⬦

SLEEP LAST NIGHT: _____ Hrs. **BEDTIME:** _____

☐ Very Good   ☐ Good   ☐ Suboptimal   ☐ Poor

TODAY'S OVERALL MOOD: 1 2 3 4 5 (HAPPIEST)

TODAY'S OVERALL STRESS: 1 2 3 4 5 (MOST STRESSED)

ADDITIONAL NOTES:

Physical Activity?

Other Symptoms?

Infections?

Menstrual Cycle?

Vitals?

Weight?

Other Habits Being Tracked?

Special Events?

*10 ounces per drop

DATE:_____   PHASE: 1   2   3

BREAKFAST / TIME_____	RESPONSE

LUNCH / TIME_____	RESPONSE

DINNER / TIME_____	RESPONSE

SNACKS / BEVERAGES	RESPONSE

REINTRODUCED FOOD (PHASE 3 ONLY): _____

BOWEL MOVEMENTS		
TIME	TYPE	NOTES

VITAMIN / MEDICATION	DOSAGE	TIME

H2O* ○ ○ ○ ○ ○ ○ ○ ○ ○ ○

SLEEP LAST NIGHT: _____ Hrs. **BEDTIME:** _____

☐ Very Good ☐ Good ☐ Suboptimal ☐ Poor

TODAY'S OVERALL MOOD: 1 2 3 4 5 (HAPPIEST)

TODAY'S OVERALL STRESS: 1 2 3 4 5 (MOST STRESSED)

ADDITIONAL NOTES:

Physical Activity?

Other Symptoms?

Infections?

Menstrual Cycle?

Vitals?

Weight?

Other Habits Being Tracked?

· Special Events?

*10 ounces per drop

55

DATE:_____ PHASE: 1   2   3

BREAKFAST / TIME_____	RESPONSE

LUNCH / TIME_____	RESPONSE

DINNER / TIME_____	RESPONSE

SNACKS / BEVERAGES	RESPONSE

REINTRODUCED FOOD (PHASE 3 ONLY): _____

BOWEL MOVEMENTS		
TIME	**TYPE**	**NOTES**

VITAMIN / MEDICATION	DOSAGE	TIME

H2O* ⬦ ⬦ ⬦ ⬦ ⬦ ⬦ ⬦ ⬦ ⬦ ⬦

SLEEP LAST NIGHT: _____ Hrs. **BEDTIME:** _____

☐ Very Good   ☐ Good   ☐ Suboptimal   ☐ Poor

TODAY'S OVERALL MOOD: 1 2 3 4 5 (HAPPIEST)

TODAY'S OVERALL STRESS: 1 2 3 4 5 (MOST STRESSED)

ADDITIONAL NOTES:

Physical Activity?

Other Symptoms?

Infections?

Menstrual Cycle?

Vitals?

Weight?

Other Habits Being
Tracked?

Special Events?

*10 ounces per drop

57

DATE:_____   PHASE: 1   2   3

BREAKFAST / TIME _____	RESPONSE

LUNCH / TIME _____	RESPONSE

DINNER / TIME _____	RESPONSE

SNACKS / BEVERAGES	RESPONSE

REINTRODUCED FOOD (PHASE 3 ONLY): _____

BOWEL MOVEMENTS		
TIME	TYPE	NOTES

VITAMIN / MEDICATION	DOSAGE	TIME

H2O* ⬡ ⬡ ⬡ ⬡ ⬡ ⬡ ⬡ ⬡ ⬡ ⬡

SLEEP LAST NIGHT: _____ Hrs. **BEDTIME:** _____

☐ Very Good ☐ Good ☐ Suboptimal ☐ Poor

TODAY'S OVERALL MOOD: 1 2 3 4 5 (HAPPIEST)

TODAY'S OVERALL STRESS: 1 2 3 4 5 (MOST STRESSED)

ADDITIONAL NOTES:

Physical Activity?

Other Symptoms?

Infections?

Menstrual Cycle?

Vitals?

Weight?

Other Habits Being Tracked?

Special Events?

*10 ounces per drop

DATE:_____   PHASE: 1   2   3

BREAKFAST / TIME_____	RESPONSE

LUNCH / TIME_____	RESPONSE

DINNER / TIME_____	RESPONSE

SNACKS / BEVERAGES	RESPONSE

REINTRODUCED FOOD (PHASE 3 ONLY): _____

BOWEL MOVEMENTS		
TIME	TYPE	NOTES

VITAMIN / MEDICATION	DOSAGE	TIME

H2O*   ⬦   ⬦   ⬦   ⬦   ⬦   ⬦   ⬦   ⬦   ⬦   ⬦

SLEEP LAST NIGHT: _____ Hrs. **BEDTIME:** _____

☐ Very Good   ☐ Good   ☐ Suboptimal   ☐ Poor

TODAY'S OVERALL MOOD: 1 2 3 4 5 (HAPPIEST)

TODAY'S OVERALL STRESS: 1 2 3 4 5 (MOST STRESSED)

ADDITIONAL NOTES:

Physical Activity?

Other Symptoms?

Infections?

Menstrual Cycle?

Vitals?

Weight?

Other Habits Being
Tracked?

Special Events?

*10 ounces per drop

DATE:_____ PHASE: 1   2   3

BREAKFAST / TIME_____	RESPONSE

LUNCH / TIME_____	RESPONSE

DINNER / TIME_____	RESPONSE

SNACKS / BEVERAGES	RESPONSE

REINTRODUCED FOOD (PHASE 3 ONLY): _____

BOWEL MOVEMENTS		
TIME	**TYPE**	**NOTES**

VITAMIN / MEDICATION	DOSAGE	TIME

H2O* ⬦ ⬦ ⬦ ⬦ ⬦ ⬦ ⬦ ⬦ ⬦ ⬦

SLEEP LAST NIGHT: _____ Hrs. **BEDTIME:** _____

☐ Very Good ☐ Good ☐ Suboptimal ☐ Poor

TODAY'S OVERALL MOOD: 1 2 3 4 5 (HAPPIEST)

TODAY'S OVERALL STRESS: 1 2 3 4 5 (MOST STRESSED)

ADDITIONAL NOTES:

Physical Activity?

Other Symptoms?

Infections?

Menstrual Cycle?

Vitals?

Weight?

Other Habits Being Tracked?

Special Events?

*10 ounces per drop

DATE:_____   PHASE: 1   2   3

BREAKFAST / TIME_____	RESPONSE

LUNCH / TIME_____	RESPONSE

DINNER / TIME_____	RESPONSE

SNACKS / BEVERAGES	RESPONSE

REINTRODUCED FOOD (PHASE 3 ONLY): _____

BOWEL MOVEMENTS		
TIME	TYPE	NOTES

VITAMIN / MEDICATION	DOSAGE	TIME

H2O* ⬭ ⬭ ⬭ ⬭ ⬭ ⬭ ⬭ ⬭ ⬭ ⬭

SLEEP LAST NIGHT: _____ Hrs. **BEDTIME:** _____

☐ Very Good ☐ Good ☐ Suboptimal ☐ Poor

TODAY'S OVERALL MOOD: 1 2 3 4 5 (HAPPIEST)

TODAY'S OVERALL STRESS: 1 2 3 4 5 (MOST STRESSED)

ADDITIONAL NOTES:

Physical Activity?

Other Symptoms?

Infections?

Menstrual Cycle?

Vitals?

Weight?

Other Habits Being Tracked?

Special Events?

*10 ounces per drop

65

DATE:_____ PHASE: 1   2   3

BREAKFAST / TIME_____	RESPONSE

LUNCH / TIME_____	RESPONSE

DINNER / TIME_____	RESPONSE

SNACKS / BEVERAGES	RESPONSE

REINTRODUCED FOOD (PHASE 3 ONLY): _____

BOWEL MOVEMENTS		
TIME	TYPE	NOTES
		.

VITAMIN / MEDICATION	DOSAGE	TIME

H2O* ◊ ◊ ◊ ◊ ◊ ◊ ◊ ◊ ◊ ◊

SLEEP LAST NIGHT: _____ Hrs. **BEDTIME:** _____

☐ Very Good   ☐ Good   ☐ Suboptimal   ☐ Poor

TODAY'S OVERALL MOOD: 1 2 3 4 5 (HAPPIEST)

TODAY'S OVERALL STRESS: 1 2 3 4 5 (MOST STRESSED)

ADDITIONAL NOTES:

Physical Activity?

Other Symptoms?

Infections?

Menstrual Cycle?

Vitals?

Weight?

Other Habits Being Tracked?

Special Events?

*10 ounces per drop

DATE:_____   PHASE: 1   2   3

BREAKFAST / TIME_____	RESPONSE

LUNCH / TIME_____	RESPONSE

DINNER / TIME_____	RESPONSE

SNACKS / BEVERAGES	RESPONSE

REINTRODUCED FOOD (PHASE 3 ONLY): _____

BOWEL MOVEMENTS

TIME	TYPE	NOTES

VITAMIN / MEDICATION	DOSAGE	TIME

H2O* ◊ ◊ ◊ ◊ ◊ ◊ ◊ ◊ ◊ ◊

SLEEP LAST NIGHT: _____ Hrs. **BEDTIME:** _____

☐ Very Good   ☐ Good   ☐ Suboptimal   ☐ Poor

TODAY'S OVERALL MOOD: 1 2 3 4 5 (HAPPIEST)

TODAY'S OVERALL STRESS: 1 2 3 4 5 (MOST STRESSED)

ADDITIONAL NOTES:

Physical Activity?

Other Symptoms?

Infections?

Menstrual Cycle?

Vitals?

Weight?

Other Habits Being Tracked?

Special Events?

*10 ounces per drop

DATE:_____ PHASE: 1   2   3

BREAKFAST / TIME_____	RESPONSE

LUNCH / TIME_____	RESPONSE

DINNER / TIME_____	RESPONSE

SNACKS / BEVERAGES	RESPONSE

REINTRODUCED FOOD (PHASE 3 ONLY): _____

BOWEL MOVEMENTS		
TIME	TYPE	NOTES

VITAMIN / MEDICATION	DOSAGE	TIME

H2O* ◌ ◌ ◌ ◌ ◌ ◌ ◌ ◌ ◌ ◌

SLEEP LAST NIGHT: _____ Hrs. **BEDTIME:** _____

☐ Very Good ☐ Good ☐ Suboptimal ☐ Poor

TODAY'S OVERALL MOOD: 1 2 3 4 5 (HAPPIEST)

TODAY'S OVERALL STRESS: 1 2 3 4 5 (MOST STRESSED)

ADDITIONAL NOTES:

Physical Activity?

Other Symptoms?

Infections?

Menstrual Cycle?

Vitals?

Weight?

Other Habits Being Tracked?

Special Events?

*10 ounces per drop

DATE:_____   PHASE: 1   2   3

BREAKFAST / TIME_____	RESPONSE

LUNCH / TIME_____	RESPONSE

DINNER / TIME_____	RESPONSE

SNACKS / BEVERAGES	RESPONSE

REINTRODUCED FOOD (PHASE 3 ONLY): _____

BOWEL MOVEMENTS		
TIME	TYPE	NOTES

VITAMIN / MEDICATION	DOSAGE	TIME

H2O*   ◊   ◊   ◊   ◊   ◊   ◊   ◊   ◊   ◊   ◊

SLEEP LAST NIGHT: _____ Hrs. **BEDTIME:** _____

☐ Very Good   ☐ Good   ☐ Suboptimal   ☐ Poor

TODAY'S OVERALL MOOD: 1 2 3 4 5 (HAPPIEST)

TODAY'S OVERALL STRESS: 1 2 3 4 5 (MOST STRESSED)

ADDITIONAL NOTES:

Physical Activity?

Other Symptoms?

Infections?

Menstrual Cycle?

Vitals?

Weight?

Other Habits Being
Tracked?

Special Events?

*10 ounces per drop

73

DATE:_____ PHASE: 1   2   3

BREAKFAST / TIME_____	RESPONSE

LUNCH / TIME_____	RESPONSE

DINNER / TIME_____	RESPONSE

SNACKS / BEVERAGES	RESPONSE

REINTRODUCED FOOD (PHASE 3 ONLY): _____

BOWEL MOVEMENTS		
TIME	**TYPE**	**NOTES**

VITAMIN / MEDICATION	DOSAGE	TIME

H2O* ⬦ ⬦ ⬦ ⬦ ⬦ ⬦ ⬦ ⬦ ⬦ ⬦

SLEEP LAST NIGHT: _____ Hrs. **BEDTIME:** _____

☐ Very Good ☐ Good ☐ Suboptimal ☐ Poor

TODAY'S OVERALL MOOD: 1 2 3 4 5 (HAPPIEST)

TODAY'S OVERALL STRESS: 1 2 3 4 5 (MOST STRESSED)

ADDITIONAL NOTES:

Physical Activity?

Other Symptoms?

Infections?

Menstrual Cycle?

Vitals?

Weight?

Other Habits Being Tracked?

Special Events?

*10 ounces per drop

DATE:_____   PHASE: 1   2   3

BREAKFAST / TIME _____	RESPONSE

LUNCH / TIME _____	RESPONSE

DINNER / TIME _____	RESPONSE

SNACKS / BEVERAGES	RESPONSE

REINTRODUCED FOOD (PHASE 3 ONLY): _____

BOWEL MOVEMENTS		
TIME	**TYPE**	**NOTES**

VITAMIN / MEDICATION	DOSAGE	TIME

H2O* ⬡ ⬡ ⬡ ⬡ ⬡ ⬡ ⬡ ⬡ ⬡ ⬡

SLEEP LAST NIGHT: _____ Hrs. **BEDTIME:** _____

☐ Very Good ☐ Good ☐ Suboptimal ☐ Poor

TODAY'S OVERALL MOOD: 1 2 3 4 5 (HAPPIEST)

TODAY'S OVERALL STRESS: 1 2 3 4 5 (MOST STRESSED)

ADDITIONAL NOTES:	
Physical Activity?	
Other Symptoms?	
Infections?	
Menstrual Cycle?	
Vitals?	
Weight?	
Other Habits Being Tracked?	
Special Events?	

*10 ounces per drop

DATE:_____ PHASE: 1   2   3

BREAKFAST / TIME_____	RESPONSE

LUNCH / TIME_____	RESPONSE

DINNER / TIME_____	RESPONSE

SNACKS / BEVERAGES	RESPONSE

REINTRODUCED FOOD (PHASE 3 ONLY): _____

BOWEL MOVEMENTS		
TIME	TYPE	NOTES

VITAMIN / MEDICATION	DOSAGE	TIME

H2O* ⬦ ⬦ ⬦ ⬦ ⬦ ⬦ ⬦ ⬦ ⬦ ⬦

SLEEP LAST NIGHT: _____ Hrs. **BEDTIME:** _____

☐ Very Good   ☐ Good   ☐ Suboptimal   ☐ Poor

TODAY'S OVERALL MOOD: 1 2 3 4 5   (HAPPIEST)

TODAY'S OVERALL STRESS: 1 2 3 4 5   (MOST STRESSED)

ADDITIONAL NOTES:

Physical Activity?

Other Symptoms?

Infections?

Menstrual Cycle?

Vitals?

Weight?

Other Habits Being Tracked?

Special Events?

*10 ounces per drop

DATE:_____   PHASE: 1   2   3

BREAKFAST / TIME_____	RESPONSE

LUNCH / TIME_____	RESPONSE

DINNER / TIME_____	RESPONSE

SNACKS / BEVERAGES	RESPONSE

REINTRODUCED FOOD (PHASE 3 ONLY): _____

BOWEL MOVEMENTS

TIME	TYPE	NOTES

VITAMIN / MEDICATION	DOSAGE	TIME

H2O* ◌ ◌ ◌ ◌ ◌ ◌ ◌ ◌ ◌ ◌

SLEEP LAST NIGHT: _____ Hrs. **BEDTIME:** _____

☐ Very Good   ☐ Good   ☐ Suboptimal   ☐ Poor

TODAY'S OVERALL MOOD: 1 2 3 4 5 (HAPPIEST)

TODAY'S OVERALL STRESS: 1 2 3 4 5 (MOST STRESSED)

ADDITIONAL NOTES:

Physical Activity?

Other Symptoms?

Infections?

Menstrual Cycle?

Vitals?

Weight?

Other Habits Being
Tracked?

Special Events?

*10 ounces per drop

DATE:_____ PHASE: 1   2   3

BREAKFAST / TIME_____	RESPONSE

LUNCH / TIME_____	RESPONSE

DINNER / TIME_____	RESPONSE

SNACKS / BEVERAGES	RESPONSE

REINTRODUCED FOOD (PHASE 3 ONLY): _____

BOWEL MOVEMENTS		
TIME	TYPE	NOTES

VITAMIN / MEDICATION	DOSAGE	TIME

H2O* ⬡ ⬡ ⬡ ⬡ ⬡ ⬡ ⬡ ⬡ ⬡ ⬡

SLEEP LAST NIGHT: _____ Hrs. **BEDTIME:** _____

☐ Very Good ☐ Good ☐ Suboptimal ☐ Poor

TODAY'S OVERALL MOOD: 1 2 3 4 5 (HAPPIEST)

TODAY'S OVERALL STRESS: 1 2 3 4 5 (MOST STRESSED)

ADDITIONAL NOTES:

Physical Activity?

Other Symptoms?

Infections?

Menstrual Cycle?

Vitals?

Weight?

Other Habits Being Tracked?

Special Events?

*10 ounces per drop

DATE:_____   PHASE: 1   2   3

BREAKFAST / TIME_____	RESPONSE

LUNCH / TIME_____	RESPONSE

DINNER / TIME_____	RESPONSE

SNACKS / BEVERAGES	RESPONSE

REINTRODUCED FOOD (PHASE 3 ONLY): _____

BOWEL MOVEMENTS		
TIME	TYPE	NOTES

VITAMIN / MEDICATION	DOSAGE	TIME

H2O* ◊ ◊ ◊ ◊ ◊ ◊ ◊ ◊ ◊ ◊

SLEEP LAST NIGHT: _____ Hrs. **BEDTIME:** _____

☐ Very Good ☐ Good ☐ Suboptimal ☐ Poor

TODAY'S OVERALL MOOD: 1 2 3 4 5 (HAPPIEST)

TODAY'S OVERALL STRESS: 1 2 3 4 5 (MOST STRESSED)

ADDITIONAL NOTES:

Physical Activity?

Other Symptoms?

Infections?

Menstrual Cycle?

Vitals?

Weight?

Other Habits Being Tracked?

Special Events?

*10 ounces per drop

85

DATE:_____   PHASE: 1   2   3

BREAKFAST / TIME_____	RESPONSE

LUNCH / TIME_____	RESPONSE

DINNER / TIME_____	RESPONSE

SNACKS / BEVERAGES	RESPONSE

REINTRODUCED FOOD (PHASE 3 ONLY): _____

BOWEL MOVEMENTS		
TIME	TYPE	NOTES

VITAMIN / MEDICATION	DOSAGE	TIME

H2O* ○ ○ ○ ○ ○ ○ ○ ○ ○ ○

SLEEP LAST NIGHT: _____ Hrs. **BEDTIME:** _____

☐ Very Good ☐ Good ☐ Suboptimal ☐ Poor

TODAY'S OVERALL MOOD: 1 2 3 4 5 (HAPPIEST)

TODAY'S OVERALL STRESS: 1 2 3 4 5 (MOST STRESSED)

ADDITIONAL NOTES:

Physical Activity?

Other Symptoms?

Infections?

Menstrual Cycle?

Vitals?

Weight?

Other Habits Being Tracked?

Special Events?

*10 ounces per drop

DATE:_____ PHASE: 1   2   3

BREAKFAST / TIME_____	RESPONSE

LUNCH / TIME_____	RESPONSE

DINNER / TIME_____	RESPONSE

SNACKS / BEVERAGES	RESPONSE

REINTRODUCED FOOD (PHASE 3 ONLY): _____

	BOWEL MOVEMENTS	
TIME	**TYPE**	**NOTES**

VITAMIN / MEDICATION	DOSAGE	TIME

H2O* ⬦ ⬦ ⬦ ⬦ ⬦ ⬦ ⬦ ⬦ ⬦ ⬦

SLEEP LAST NIGHT: _____ Hrs. **BEDTIME:** _____

☐ Very Good ☐ Good ☐ Suboptimal ☐ Poor

TODAY'S OVERALL MOOD: 1 2 3 4 5 (HAPPIEST)

TODAY'S OVERALL STRESS: 1 2 3 4 5 (MOST STRESSED)

ADDITIONAL NOTES:

Physical Activity?

Other Symptoms?

Infections?

Menstrual Cycle?

Vitals?

Weight?

Other Habits Being Tracked?

Special Events?

*10 ounces per drop

DATE:_____ PHASE: 1   2   3

BREAKFAST / TIME_____	RESPONSE

LUNCH / TIME_____	RESPONSE

DINNER / TIME_____	RESPONSE

SNACKS / BEVERAGES	RESPONSE

REINTRODUCED FOOD (PHASE 3 ONLY): _____

BOWEL MOVEMENTS		
TIME	**TYPE**	**NOTES**

VITAMIN / MEDICATION	DOSAGE	TIME

H2O* 　⬦　⬦　⬦　⬦　⬦　⬦　⬦　⬦　⬦　⬦

SLEEP LAST NIGHT: _____ Hrs. **BEDTIME:** _____

☐ Very Good   ☐ Good   ☐ Suboptimal   ☐ Poor

TODAY'S OVERALL MOOD:　1　2　3　4　5　(HAPPIEST)

TODAY'S OVERALL STRESS:　1　2　3　4　5　(MOST STRESSED)

ADDITIONAL NOTES:	
Physical Activity?	
Other Symptoms?	
Infections?	
Menstrual Cycle?	
Vitals?	
Weight?	
Other Habits Being Tracked?	
Special Events?	

*10 ounces per drop

DATE:_____ PHASE: 1   2   3

BREAKFAST / TIME_____	RESPONSE

LUNCH / TIME_____	RESPONSE

DINNER / TIME_____	RESPONSE

SNACKS / BEVERAGES	RESPONSE

REINTRODUCED FOOD (PHASE 3 ONLY): _____

	BOWEL MOVEMENTS	
TIME	TYPE	NOTES

VITAMIN / MEDICATION	DOSAGE	TIME

H2O*   ○   ○   ○   ○   ○   ○   ○   ○   ○   ○

SLEEP LAST NIGHT: _____ Hrs. **BEDTIME:** _____

☐ Very Good   ☐ Good   ☐ Suboptimal   ☐ Poor

TODAY'S OVERALL MOOD: 1 2 3 4 5 (HAPPIEST)

TODAY'S OVERALL STRESS: 1 2 3 4 5 (MOST STRESSED)

ADDITIONAL NOTES:

Physical Activity?

Other Symptoms?

Infections?

Menstrual Cycle?

Vitals?

Weight?

Other Habits Being Tracked?

Special Events?

*10 ounces per drop

DATE:_____ PHASE: 1   2   3

BREAKFAST / TIME_____	RESPONSE

LUNCH / TIME_____	RESPONSE

DINNER / TIME_____	RESPONSE

SNACKS / BEVERAGES	RESPONSE

REINTRODUCED FOOD (PHASE 3 ONLY): _____

BOWEL MOVEMENTS		
TIME	TYPE	NOTES

VITAMIN / MEDICATION	DOSAGE	TIME

H2O* ⬡ ⬡ ⬡ ⬡ ⬡ ⬡ ⬡ ⬡ ⬡ ⬡

SLEEP LAST NIGHT: _____ Hrs. **BEDTIME:** _____

☐ Very Good ☐ Good ☐ Suboptimal ☐ Poor

TODAY'S OVERALL MOOD: 1 2 3 4 5 (HAPPIEST)

TODAY'S OVERALL STRESS: 1 2 3 4 5 (MOST STRESSED)

ADDITIONAL NOTES:

Physical Activity?

Other Symptoms?

Infections?

Menstrual Cycle?

Vitals?

Weight?

Other Habits Being Tracked?

Special Events?

*10 ounces per drop

DATE:_____   PHASE: 1   2   3

BREAKFAST / TIME_____	RESPONSE

LUNCH / TIME_____	RESPONSE

DINNER / TIME_____	RESPONSE

SNACKS / BEVERAGES	RESPONSE

REINTRODUCED FOOD (PHASE 3 ONLY): _____

BOWEL MOVEMENTS		
TIME	TYPE	NOTES

VITAMIN / MEDICATION	DOSAGE	TIME

H2O*   ○   ○   ○   ○   ○   ○   ○   ○   ○   ○

SLEEP LAST NIGHT: _____ Hrs. **BEDTIME:** _____

☐ Very Good   ☐ Good   ☐ Suboptimal   ☐ Poor

TODAY'S OVERALL MOOD: 1 2 3 4 5 (HAPPIEST)

TODAY'S OVERALL STRESS: 1 2 3 4 5 (MOST STRESSED)

ADDITIONAL NOTES:

Physical Activity?

Other Symptoms?

Infections?

Menstrual Cycle?

Vitals?

Weight?

Other Habits Being
Tracked?

Special Events?

*10 ounces per drop

DATE:_____   PHASE: 1   2   3

BREAKFAST / TIME_____	RESPONSE

LUNCH / TIME_____	RESPONSE

DINNER / TIME_____	RESPONSE

SNACKS / BEVERAGES	RESPONSE

REINTRODUCED FOOD (PHASE 3 ONLY): _____

BOWEL MOVEMENTS		
TIME	TYPE	NOTES

VITAMIN / MEDICATION	DOSAGE	TIME

H2O*   ◌   ◌   ◌   ◌   ◌   ◌   ◌   ◌   ◌   ◌

SLEEP LAST NIGHT: _____ Hrs. **BEDTIME:** _____

☐ Very Good   ☐ Good   ☐ Suboptimal   ☐ Poor

TODAY'S OVERALL MOOD: 1 2 3 4 5 (HAPPIEST)

TODAY'S OVERALL STRESS: 1 2 3 4 5 (MOST STRESSED)

ADDITIONAL NOTES:

Physical Activity?

Other Symptoms?

Infections?

Menstrual Cycle?

Vitals?

Weight?

Other Habits Being
Tracked?

Special Events?

*10 ounces per drop

DATE:_____   PHASE: 1   2   3

BREAKFAST / TIME _____	RESPONSE

LUNCH / TIME _____	RESPONSE

DINNER / TIME _____	RESPONSE

SNACKS / BEVERAGES	RESPONSE

REINTRODUCED FOOD (PHASE 3 ONLY): _____

BOWEL MOVEMENTS		
TIME	**TYPE**	**NOTES**

VITAMIN / MEDICATION	DOSAGE	TIME

H2O*   ⬠ ⬠ ⬠ ⬠ ⬠ ⬠ ⬠ ⬠ ⬠ ⬠

SLEEP LAST NIGHT: _____ Hrs. **BEDTIME:** _____

☐ Very Good   ☐ Good   ☐ Suboptimal   ☐ Poor

TODAY'S OVERALL MOOD: 1 2 3 4 5 (HAPPIEST)

TODAY'S OVERALL STRESS: 1 2 3 4 5 (MOST STRESSED)

ADDITIONAL NOTES:

Physical Activity?

Other Symptoms?

Infections?

Menstrual Cycle?

Vitals?

Weight?

Other Habits Being Tracked?

Special Events?

*10 ounces per drop

DATE:_____   PHASE: 1   2   3

BREAKFAST / TIME_____	RESPONSE

LUNCH / TIME_____	RESPONSE

DINNER / TIME_____	RESPONSE

SNACKS / BEVERAGES	RESPONSE

REINTRODUCED FOOD (PHASE 3 ONLY): _____

BOWEL MOVEMENTS		
TIME	TYPE	NOTES

VITAMIN / MEDICATION	DOSAGE	TIME

H2O* ⬦ ⬦ ⬦ ⬦ ⬦ ⬦ ⬦ ⬦ ⬦ ⬦

SLEEP LAST NIGHT: _____ Hrs. **BEDTIME:** _____

☐ Very Good   ☐ Good   ☐ Suboptimal   ☐ Poor

TODAY'S OVERALL MOOD: 1 2 3 4 5 (HAPPIEST)

TODAY'S OVERALL STRESS: 1 2 3 4 5 (MOST STRESSED)

ADDITIONAL NOTES:

Physical Activity?

Other Symptoms?

Infections?

Menstrual Cycle?

Vitals?

Weight?

Other Habits Being
Tracked?

Special Events?

*10 ounces per drop

DATE:_____   PHASE: 1   2   3

BREAKFAST / TIME_____	RESPONSE

LUNCH / TIME_____	RESPONSE

DINNER / TIME_____	RESPONSE

SNACKS / BEVERAGES	RESPONSE

REINTRODUCED FOOD (PHASE 3 ONLY): _____

BOWEL MOVEMENTS		
TIME	TYPE	NOTES

VITAMIN / MEDICATION	DOSAGE	TIME

H2O* ◊ ◊ ◊ ◊ ◊ ◊ ◊ ◊ ◊ ◊

SLEEP LAST NIGHT: _____ Hrs. **BEDTIME:** _____

☐ Very Good   ☐ Good   ☐ Suboptimal   ☐ Poor

TODAY'S OVERALL MOOD: 1 2 3 4 5 (HAPPIEST)

TODAY'S OVERALL STRESS: 1 2 3 4 5 (MOST STRESSED)

ADDITIONAL NOTES:	
Physical Activity?	
Other Symptoms?	
Infections?	
Menstrual Cycle?	
Vitals?	
Weight?	
Other Habits Being Tracked?	
Special Events?	

*10 ounces per drop

DATE:_____   PHASE: 1   2   3

BREAKFAST / TIME_____	RESPONSE

LUNCH / TIME_____	RESPONSE

DINNER / TIME_____	RESPONSE

SNACKS / BEVERAGES	RESPONSE

REINTRODUCED FOOD (PHASE 3 ONLY): _____

BOWEL MOVEMENTS		
TIME	TYPE	NOTES

VITAMIN / MEDICATION	DOSAGE	TIME

H2O*   ◊ ◊ ◊ ◊ ◊ ◊ ◊ ◊ ◊ ◊

SLEEP LAST NIGHT: _____ Hrs. **BEDTIME:** _____

☐ Very Good   ☐ Good   ☐ Suboptimal   ☐ Poor

TODAY'S OVERALL MOOD: 1 2 3 4 5 (HAPPIEST)

TODAY'S OVERALL STRESS: 1 2 3 4 5 (MOST STRESSED)

ADDITIONAL NOTES:	
Physical Activity?	
Other Symptoms?	
Infections?	
Menstrual Cycle?	
Vitals?	
Weight?	
Other Habits Being Tracked?	
Special Events?	

*10 ounces per drop

DATE:_____ PHASE: 1   2   3

BREAKFAST / TIME_____	RESPONSE

LUNCH / TIME_____	RESPONSE

DINNER / TIME_____	RESPONSE

SNACKS / BEVERAGES	RESPONSE

REINTRODUCED FOOD (PHASE 3 ONLY): _____

BOWEL MOVEMENTS		
TIME	**TYPE**	**NOTES**

VITAMIN / MEDICATION	DOSAGE	TIME

H2O* ○ ○ ○ ○ ○ ○ ○ ○ ○ ○

SLEEP LAST NIGHT: _____ Hrs. **BEDTIME:** _____

☐ Very Good ☐ Good ☐ Suboptimal ☐ Poor

TODAY'S OVERALL MOOD: 1 2 3 4 5 (HAPPIEST)

TODAY'S OVERALL STRESS: 1 2 3 4 5 (MOST STRESSED)

ADDITIONAL NOTES:

Physical Activity?

Other Symptoms?

Infections?

Menstrual Cycle?

Vitals?

Weight?

Other Habits Being Tracked?

Special Events?

*10 ounces per drop

DATE:_____ PHASE: 1   2   3

BREAKFAST / TIME_____	RESPONSE

LUNCH / TIME_____	RESPONSE

DINNER / TIME_____	RESPONSE

SNACKS / BEVERAGES	RESPONSE

REINTRODUCED FOOD (PHASE 3 ONLY): _____

BOWEL MOVEMENTS

TIME	TYPE	NOTES

VITAMIN / MEDICATION	DOSAGE	TIME

H2O* ◊ ◊ ◊ ◊ ◊ ◊ ◊ ◊ ◊ ◊

SLEEP LAST NIGHT: _____ Hrs. **BEDTIME:** _____

☐ Very Good   ☐ Good   ☐ Suboptimal   ☐ Poor

TODAY'S OVERALL MOOD: 1 2 3 4 5 (HAPPIEST)

TODAY'S OVERALL STRESS: 1 2 3 4 5 (MOST STRESSED)

ADDITIONAL NOTES:

Physical Activity?

Other Symptoms?

Infections?

Menstrual Cycle?

Vitals?

Weight?

Other Habits Being
Tracked?

Special Events?

*10 ounces per drop

DATE:_____   PHASE: 1   2   3

BREAKFAST / TIME_____	RESPONSE

LUNCH / TIME_____	RESPONSE

DINNER / TIME_____	RESPONSE

SNACKS / BEVERAGES	RESPONSE

REINTRODUCED FOOD (PHASE 3 ONLY): _____

BOWEL MOVEMENTS		
TIME	TYPE	NOTES

VITAMIN / MEDICATION	DOSAGE	TIME

H2O*   ◊   ◊   ◊   ◊   ◊   ◊   ◊   ◊   ◊   ◊

SLEEP LAST NIGHT: _____ Hrs. **BEDTIME:** _____

☐ Very Good   ☐ Good   ☐ Suboptimal   ☐ Poor

TODAY'S OVERALL MOOD: 1 2 3 4 5   (HAPPIEST)

TODAY'S OVERALL STRESS: 1 2 3 4 5   (MOST STRESSED)

ADDITIONAL NOTES:

Physical Activity?

Other Symptoms?

Infections?

Menstrual Cycle?

Vitals?

Weight?

Other Habits Being
Tracked?

Special Events?

*10 ounces per drop

DATE:_____   PHASE: 1   2   3

BREAKFAST / TIME_____	RESPONSE

LUNCH / TIME_____	RESPONSE

DINNER / TIME_____	RESPONSE

SNACKS / BEVERAGES	RESPONSE

REINTRODUCED FOOD (PHASE 3 ONLY): _____

BOWEL MOVEMENTS		
TIME	TYPE	NOTES

VITAMIN / MEDICATION	DOSAGE	TIME

H2O* ⬦ ⬦ ⬦ ⬦ ⬦ ⬦ ⬦ ⬦ ⬦ ⬦

SLEEP LAST NIGHT: _____ Hrs. **BEDTIME:** _____

☐ Very Good ☐ Good ☐ Suboptimal ☐ Poor

TODAY'S OVERALL MOOD: 1 2 3 4 5 (HAPPIEST)

TODAY'S OVERALL STRESS: 1 2 3 4 5 (MOST STRESSED)

ADDITIONAL NOTES:

Physical Activity?

Other Symptoms?

Infections?

Menstrual Cycle?

Vitals?

Weight?

Other Habits Being Tracked?

Special Events?

*10 ounces per drop

DATE:_____ PHASE: 1   2   3

BREAKFAST / TIME_____	RESPONSE

LUNCH / TIME_____	RESPONSE

DINNER / TIME_____	RESPONSE

SNACKS / BEVERAGES	RESPONSE

REINTRODUCED FOOD (PHASE 3 ONLY): _____

BOWEL MOVEMENTS		
TIME	TYPE	NOTES

VITAMIN / MEDICATION	DOSAGE	TIME

H2O*   ⬡   ⬡   ⬡   ⬡   ⬡   ⬡   ⬡   ⬡   ⬡   ⬡

SLEEP LAST NIGHT: _____ Hrs. **BEDTIME:** _____

☐ Very Good   ☐ Good   ☐ Suboptimal   ☐ Poor

TODAY'S OVERALL MOOD: 1 2 3 4 5 (HAPPIEST)

TODAY'S OVERALL STRESS: 1 2 3 4 5 (MOST STRESSED)

ADDITIONAL NOTES:

Physical Activity?

Other Symptoms?

Infections?

Menstrual Cycle?

Vitals?

Weight?

Other Habits Being
Tracked?

Special Events?

*10 ounces per drop

DATE:_____   PHASE: 1   2   3

BREAKFAST / TIME _____	RESPONSE

LUNCH / TIME _____	RESPONSE

DINNER / TIME _____	RESPONSE

SNACKS / BEVERAGES	RESPONSE

REINTRODUCED FOOD (PHASE 3 ONLY): _____

BOWEL MOVEMENTS		
TIME	TYPE	NOTES

VITAMIN / MEDICATION	DOSAGE	TIME

H2O*   ○   ○   ○   ○   ○   ○   ○   ○   ○   ○

SLEEP LAST NIGHT: _____ Hrs. **BEDTIME:** _____

☐ Very Good   ☐ Good   ☐ Suboptimal   ☐ Poor

TODAY'S OVERALL MOOD: 1   2   3   4   5   (HAPPIEST)

TODAY'S OVERALL STRESS: 1   2   3   4   5   (MOST STRESSED)

ADDITIONAL NOTES:

Physical Activity?

Other Symptoms?

Infections?

Menstrual Cycle?

Vitals?

Weight?

Other Habits Being Tracked?

Special Events?

*10 ounces per drop

DATE:_____ PHASE: 1   2   3

BREAKFAST / TIME_____	RESPONSE

LUNCH / TIME_____	RESPONSE

DINNER / TIME_____	RESPONSE

SNACKS / BEVERAGES	RESPONSE

REINTRODUCED FOOD (PHASE 3 ONLY): _____

BOWEL MOVEMENTS		
TIME	TYPE	NOTES

VITAMIN / MEDICATION	DOSAGE	TIME

H2O* ⬦ ⬦ ⬦ ⬦ ⬦ ⬦ ⬦ ⬦ ⬦ ⬦

SLEEP LAST NIGHT: _____ Hrs. **BEDTIME:** _____

☐ Very Good   ☐ Good   ☐ Suboptimal   ☐ Poor

TODAY'S OVERALL MOOD: 1 2 3 4 5 (HAPPIEST)

TODAY'S OVERALL STRESS: 1 2 3 4 5 (MOST STRESSED)

ADDITIONAL NOTES:

Physical Activity?

Other Symptoms?

Infections?

Menstrual Cycle?

Vitals?

Weight?

Other Habits Being Tracked?

Special Events?

*10 ounces per drop

DATE:_____ PHASE: 1   2   3

BREAKFAST / TIME_____	RESPONSE

LUNCH / TIME_____	RESPONSE

DINNER / TIME_____	RESPONSE

SNACKS / BEVERAGES	RESPONSE

REINTRODUCED FOOD (PHASE 3 ONLY): _____

BOWEL MOVEMENTS

TIME	TYPE	NOTES

VITAMIN / MEDICATION	DOSAGE	TIME

H2O*   ⬡ ⬡ ⬡ ⬡ ⬡ ⬡ ⬡ ⬡ ⬡ ⬡

SLEEP LAST NIGHT: _____ Hrs. **BEDTIME:** _____

☐ Very Good   ☐ Good   ☐ Suboptimal   ☐ Poor

TODAY'S OVERALL MOOD: 1 2 3 4 5   (HAPPIEST)

TODAY'S OVERALL STRESS: 1 2 3 4 5   (MOST STRESSED)

ADDITIONAL NOTES:

Physical Activity?

Other Symptoms?

Infections?

Menstrual Cycle?

Vitals?

Weight?

Other Habits Being
Tracked?

Special Events?

*10 ounces per drop

DATE:_____   PHASE: 1   2   3

BREAKFAST / TIME_____	RESPONSE

LUNCH / TIME_____	RESPONSE

DINNER / TIME_____	RESPONSE

SNACKS / BEVERAGES	RESPONSE

REINTRODUCED FOOD (PHASE 3 ONLY): _____

BOWEL MOVEMENTS

TIME	TYPE	NOTES

VITAMIN / MEDICATION	DOSAGE	TIME

H2O* ⬦ ⬦ ⬦ ⬦ ⬦ ⬦ ⬦ ⬦ ⬦ ⬦

SLEEP LAST NIGHT: _____ Hrs. **BEDTIME:** _____

☐ Very Good ☐ Good ☐ Suboptimal ☐ Poor

TODAY'S OVERALL MOOD: 1 2 3 4 5 (HAPPIEST)

TODAY'S OVERALL STRESS: 1 2 3 4 5 (MOST STRESSED)

ADDITIONAL NOTES:

Physical Activity?

Other Symptoms?

Infections?

Menstrual Cycle?

Vitals?

Weight?

Other Habits Being Tracked?

Special Events?

*10 ounces per drop

DATE:_____   PHASE: 1   2   3

BREAKFAST / TIME_____	RESPONSE

LUNCH / TIME_____	RESPONSE

DINNER / TIME_____	RESPONSE

SNACKS / BEVERAGES	RESPONSE

REINTRODUCED FOOD (PHASE 3 ONLY): _____

BOWEL MOVEMENTS		
TIME	TYPE	NOTES

VITAMIN / MEDICATION	DOSAGE	TIME

H2O* ⬠ ⬠ ⬠ ⬠ ⬠ ⬠ ⬠ ⬠ ⬠ ⬠

SLEEP LAST NIGHT: _____ Hrs. **BEDTIME:** _____

☐ Very Good   ☐ Good   ☐ Suboptimal   ☐ Poor

TODAY'S OVERALL MOOD: 1 2 3 4 5 (HAPPIEST)

TODAY'S OVERALL STRESS: 1 2 3 4 5 (MOST STRESSED)

ADDITIONAL NOTES:

Physical Activity?

Other Symptoms?

Infections?

Menstrual Cycle?

Vitals?

Weight?

Other Habits Being Tracked?

Special Events?

*10 ounces per drop

DATE:_____   PHASE: 1   2   3

BREAKFAST / TIME_____	RESPONSE

LUNCH / TIME_____	RESPONSE

DINNER / TIME_____	RESPONSE

SNACKS / BEVERAGES	RESPONSE

REINTRODUCED FOOD (PHASE 3 ONLY): _____

BOWEL MOVEMENTS		
TIME	TYPE	NOTES

VITAMIN / MEDICATION	DOSAGE	TIME

H2O* ◊ ◊ ◊ ◊ ◊ ◊ ◊ ◊ ◊ ◊

SLEEP LAST NIGHT: _____ Hrs. **BEDTIME:** _____

☐ Very Good ☐ Good ☐ Suboptimal ☐ Poor

TODAY'S OVERALL MOOD: 1 2 3 4 5 (HAPPIEST)

TODAY'S OVERALL STRESS: 1 2 3 4 5 (MOST STRESSED)

ADDITIONAL NOTES:

Physical Activity?

Other Symptoms?

Infections?

Menstrual Cycle?

Vitals?

Weight?

Other Habits Being Tracked?

Special Events?

*10 ounces per drop

DATE:_____ PHASE: 1   2   3

BREAKFAST / TIME_____	RESPONSE

LUNCH / TIME_____	RESPONSE

DINNER / TIME_____	RESPONSE

SNACKS / BEVERAGES	RESPONSE

REINTRODUCED FOOD (PHASE 3 ONLY): _____

BOWEL MOVEMENTS		
TIME	**TYPE**	**NOTES**

VITAMIN / MEDICATION	DOSAGE	TIME

H2O* ○ ○ ○ ○ ○ ○ ○ ○ ○ ○

SLEEP LAST NIGHT: _____ Hrs. **BEDTIME:** _____

☐ Very Good   ☐ Good   ☐ Suboptimal   ☐ Poor

TODAY'S OVERALL MOOD: 1 2 3 4 5 (HAPPIEST)

TODAY'S OVERALL STRESS: 1 2 3 4 5 (MOST STRESSED)

ADDITIONAL NOTES:	
Physical Activity?	
Other Symptoms?	
Infections?	
Menstrual Cycle?	
Vitals?	
Weight?	
Other Habits Being Tracked?	
Special Events?	

*10 ounces per drop

DATE:_____ PHASE: 1   2   3

BREAKFAST / TIME_____	RESPONSE

LUNCH / TIME_____	RESPONSE

DINNER / TIME_____	RESPONSE

SNACKS / BEVERAGES	RESPONSE

REINTRODUCED FOOD (PHASE 3 ONLY): _____

	BOWEL MOVEMENTS	
TIME	TYPE	NOTES

VITAMIN / MEDICATION	DOSAGE	TIME

H2O* ○ ○ ○ ○ ○ ○ ○ ○ ○ ○

SLEEP LAST NIGHT: _____ Hrs. **BEDTIME:** _____

☐ Very Good ☐ Good ☐ Suboptimal ☐ Poor

TODAY'S OVERALL MOOD: 1 2 3 4 5 (HAPPIEST)

TODAY'S OVERALL STRESS: 1 2 3 4 5 (MOST STRESSED)

ADDITIONAL NOTES:

Physical Activity?

Other Symptoms?

Infections?

Menstrual Cycle?

Vitals?

Weight?

Other Habits Being Tracked?

Special Events?

*10 ounces per drop

DATE:_____ PHASE: 1   2   3

BREAKFAST / TIME_____	RESPONSE

LUNCH / TIME_____	RESPONSE

DINNER / TIME_____	RESPONSE

SNACKS / BEVERAGES	RESPONSE

REINTRODUCED FOOD (PHASE 3 ONLY): _____

BOWEL MOVEMENTS		
TIME	TYPE	NOTES

VITAMIN / MEDICATION	DOSAGE	TIME

H2O* ○ ○ ○ ○ ○ ○ ○ ○ ○ ○

SLEEP LAST NIGHT: _____ Hrs. **BEDTIME:** _____

☐ Very Good ☐ Good ☐ Suboptimal ☐ Poor

TODAY'S OVERALL MOOD: 1 2 3 4 5 (HAPPIEST)

TODAY'S OVERALL STRESS: 1 2 3 4 5 (MOST STRESSED)

ADDITIONAL NOTES:	
Physical Activity?	
Other Symptoms?	
Infections?	
Menstrual Cycle?	
Vitals?	
Weight?	
Other Habits Being Tracked?	
Special Events?	

*10 ounces per drop

DATE:_____   PHASE: 1   2   3

BREAKFAST / TIME_____	RESPONSE

LUNCH / TIME_____	RESPONSE

DINNER / TIME_____	RESPONSE

SNACKS / BEVERAGES	RESPONSE

REINTRODUCED FOOD (PHASE 3 ONLY): _____

BOWEL MOVEMENTS

TIME	TYPE	NOTES

VITAMIN / MEDICATION	DOSAGE	TIME

H2O* ◊ ◊ ◊ ◊ ◊ ◊ ◊ ◊ ◊ ◊

SLEEP LAST NIGHT: _____ Hrs. **BEDTIME:** _____

☐ Very Good   ☐ Good   ☐ Suboptimal   ☐ Poor

TODAY'S OVERALL MOOD: 1 2 3 4 5 (HAPPIEST)

TODAY'S OVERALL STRESS: 1 2 3 4 5 (MOST STRESSED)

ADDITIONAL NOTES:

Physical Activity?

Other Symptoms?

Infections?

Menstrual Cycle?

Vitals?

Weight?

Other Habits Being Tracked?

Special Events?

*10 ounces per drop

DATE:_____   PHASE: 1   2   3

BREAKFAST / TIME_____	RESPONSE

LUNCH / TIME_____	RESPONSE

DINNER / TIME_____	RESPONSE

SNACKS / BEVERAGES	RESPONSE

REINTRODUCED FOOD (PHASE 3 ONLY): _____

BOWEL MOVEMENTS

TIME	TYPE	NOTES

VITAMIN / MEDICATION	DOSAGE	TIME

H2O*   ◊   ◊   ◊   ◊   ◊   ◊   ◊   ◊   ◊   ◊

SLEEP LAST NIGHT: _____ Hrs. **BEDTIME:** _____

☐ Very Good   ☐ Good   ☐ Suboptimal   ☐ Poor

TODAY'S OVERALL MOOD: 1 2 3 4 5 (HAPPIEST)

TODAY'S OVERALL STRESS: 1 2 3 4 5 (MOST STRESSED)

ADDITIONAL NOTES:

Physical Activity?

Other Symptoms?

Infections?

Menstrual Cycle?

Vitals?

Weight?

Other Habits Being Tracked?

Special Events?

*10 ounces per drop

DATE:_____   PHASE: 1   2   3

BREAKFAST / TIME_____	RESPONSE

LUNCH / TIME_____	RESPONSE

DINNER / TIME_____	RESPONSE

SNACKS / BEVERAGES	RESPONSE

REINTRODUCED FOOD (PHASE 3 ONLY): _____

BOWEL MOVEMENTS		
TIME	**TYPE**	**NOTES**

VITAMIN / MEDICATION	DOSAGE	TIME

H2O* ◊ ◊ ◊ ◊ ◊ ◊ ◊ ◊ ◊ ◊

SLEEP LAST NIGHT: _____ Hrs. **BEDTIME:** _____

☐ Very Good   ☐ Good   ☐ Suboptimal   ☐ Poor

TODAY'S OVERALL MOOD: 1 2 3 4 5 (HAPPIEST)

TODAY'S OVERALL STRESS: 1 2 3 4 5 (MOST STRESSED)

ADDITIONAL NOTES:	
Physical Activity?	
Other Symptoms?	
Infections?	
Menstrual Cycle?	
Vitals?	
Weight?	
Other Habits Being Tracked?	
Special Events?	

*10 ounces per drop

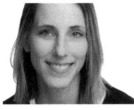

Heidi Moretti, MS, RD, is a writer and author of the book *The Whole-Body Guide to Gut Health* and the website The Healthy RD. She has been a practicing clinical registered dietitian for 22 years, much of that with Providence St. Patrick Hospital and in the last couple years with Fresenius Kidney Care. Heidi has a passion for putting more healing into medicine by using functional nutrition, holistic health, and natural medicine to get to the root causes of illnesses.

Heidi received a master of science in nutritional science from the University of Washington. She has a passion for improving vitality through food. When Heidi was pursuing her undergraduate studies at Montana State University, she developed her love of nutrition and became inspired to pursue her career path.

Heidi has researched vitamins, supplements, and food as medicine throughout her career, and her research has been published in peer-reviewed journals like the *Journal of Renal Nutrition* and *BMC Cardiovascular Disorders*.